American Health – Who Gets Paid

Robin Blackstone, MD

Blackstone Press

Published by Blackstone Press.

ISBN: 979-8-9940978-4-7 **(Paperback)**

This short book is written for people working in health care who sense that something fundamental has changed but have not yet been given clear language for it. It is intended to be read in parts, discussed, and tested locally. No prior agreement is assumed.

Printed in the United States of America.

Introduction: The Money Machine

Most American physicians believe that payment follows the care they provide—that time spent with patients, judgment applied under uncertainty, and responsibility carried when things go wrong are, in some reasonable way, reflected in how they are paid. They may not like the details, but they assume the system broadly mirrors their work.

It does not.

What determines how doctors are paid in the United States is not a market in any ordinary sense, nor a public budget debated in the open. It is a private pricing system, built over decades, maintained largely out of view, and enforced through rules so technical that even those who depend on them rarely see the full structure.

That structure governs far more than income. It shapes how long physicians spend with patients, which kinds of care are encouraged, which are postponed, and which quietly disappear. It rewards certain actions and penalizes others. And because it operates behind the scenes, it is almost never questioned by those most affected by it.

Physicians do not control this system. Patients do not see it. Employers pay into it without understanding it. Policymakers gesture toward reform while missing its core mechanics. Yet this machinery quietly dictates how American medicine is practiced, day after day, exam room by exam room.

To understand how this happened, we need to be precise about terms that are often used loosely—or not explained at all.

At the center of the system are CPT codes, short for Current Procedural Terminology. Despite the name, these codes are not simply a list of procedures. They form the official billing language of American medicine. Nearly every billable act—from a complex surgery to a brief office visit—must be translated into this code set. Care that cannot be described in this language cannot be paid for.

Each CPT code is assigned a numerical value called an RVU, or Relative Value Unit. An RVU is intended to represent how much a service is "worth" compared to others. In theory, it reflects time, effort, training, and risk. In practice, it functions as a pricing unit. Higher RVUs lead to higher payment.

Who assigns those values?

That task falls largely to the Relative Value Scale Update Committee, known as the RUC. The RUC is convened by the American Medical Association, a private professional organization. Its members are primarily physicians appointed through specialty societies. The committee meets behind closed doors to recommend how much each service should be worth.

Those recommendations are then transmitted to the federal government, which adopts the vast majority of them—not because they are beyond dispute, but because no alternative pricing system exists to replace them. The government lacks an independent apparatus capable of valuing medical work at this scale. The result is structural dependence.

The composition of the RUC therefore matters. Specialty societies representing procedure-based fields make up a substantial share of the committee. It stands to reason that services requiring more equipment, personnel, and billable activity tend to be valued more highly than services that rely primarily on time, judgment, explanation, or continuity of care.

This arrangement is often described as

technical or neutral. In reality, it is a form of governance—meaning a system that determines who decides, by what rules, and with what consequences. It is one of the most influential governance structures in American health care, and one of the least examined.

The effects are visible. Procedural intervention is rewarded. Prevention is discounted. Longitudinal care is squeezed. Thinking work loses ground to doing work. Over time, the system has come to favor activity over outcomes and volume over health.

None of this was inevitable. The system was built for a different era of medicine—one dominated by acute illness, hospital-based care, and discrete interventions. It assumed that prevention would be secondary, that chronic disease would be managed episodically, and that meaningful work would occur within institutional walls.

Those assumptions no longer hold.

Medicine today revolves around chronic conditions, long time horizons, and continuous management. Digital tools allow monitoring, guidance, and coordination to occur far from hospitals. Patients live with disease rather than passing briefly through it. Yet the pricing system remains anchored to an older logic, enforcing priorities that no longer match clinical reality.

The problem is often described as one of incentives—a word that simply means what the system makes easier or harder to do. But incentives do not arise by accident. They are the result of design choices, embedded in rules, and sustained by institutions that benefit from their continuation.

This book examines how those choices were made, how they hardened into habit, and why they now stand in the way of better health. It does not argue that physicians are greedy, that policymakers are foolish, or that patients expect too much. It argues something more uncomfortable: that American medicine is governed by a pricing system that no longer serves its stated purpose.

Physicians deserve to understand the system that shapes their work. Patients deserve to know why care so often feels misaligned with their needs. And the country deserves a way of paying for medicine that rewards health, not just intervention.

Chapter 1: What Gets Paid For Gets Done

Every system reveals its priorities through what it rewards.

In American medicine, the reward is not health. It is activity.

This is not a moral judgment. It is an operational fact. Professionals respond, as they always have, to the conditions under which they work. When payment favors certain forms of work over others, behavior follows. When time is undervalued, visits shorten. When continuity goes unpaid, it weakens. When prevention is poorly rewarded, it recedes.

These outcomes are often described as unintended side effects. In fact, they are predictable results of the pricing structure itself.

Consider the work that occupies much

of modern medicine. A physician listens to a patient describe symptoms that do not fit neatly into categories. She weighs incomplete information, considers tradeoffs, explains uncertainty, and helps the patient decide what to do next. She may also take responsibility for checking in later, adjusting the plan, and noticing when something subtle changes.

This work requires training and judgment. It depends on trust built over time. And it involves accountability—not in the sense of blame, but in the sense of sustained responsibility for guiding health across months or years.

Yet in the prevailing payment system, this work is compressed into narrow billing categories with limited value. It is treated as brief, interchangeable, and easily substituted, regardless of complexity.

By contrast, procedural intervention fits cleanly into the billing framework.

Procedures can be scheduled, timed, staffed, documented, and counted. They use equipment. They involve multiple people. They generate records that are easy to audit. As a result, they are easier to price—and they are priced higher.

The bias is structural, not personal. The system favors what it can count.

Over time, this logic compounds. Practices adapt. Staffing models change. Appointment slots shrink. Longitudinal problem-solving is pushed to the margins. Physicians learn, often unconsciously, which forms of work sustain a practice and which quietly drain time and energy.

Patients experience the result as fragmentation. They see multiple clinicians, repeat their story, and receive guidance that feels rushed or incomplete. Employers experience it as rising costs without clear gains in health. Policymakers experience it as a cycle of reform efforts that never seem to reach the core of the problem.

The language of "incentives" often obscures what is really happening. Incentives sound abstract, even optional. In practice, they function more like gravity. They shape behavior steadily and relentlessly, regardless of individual intention.

This gravity is reinforced by governance. The bodies that assign value to medical work are composed of people whose own experience shapes what they see as legitimate effort. A pricing committee dominated by procedure-based specialties will, quite naturally, prize procedures. A committee dominated by longitudinal generalists would almost certainly price differently. Either way, the composition matters because it determines what the system treats as real work.

Appeals to professionalism cannot correct this imbalance on their own. Clinicians still have payrolls, leases, and families. A system that pays poorly for upstream work will, over time, drive that work out of the system, no matter how dedicated the professionals within it may be.

As upstream intervention becomes more effective—through better data, earlier signals, and continuous monitoring—the current premium placed on late rescue will begin to look less like tradition and more like mispricing. The institutions that benefit most from today's arrangement will try to preserve it. Any serious reform must offer them a credible alternative rather than a moral rebuke.

As long as the underlying pricing logic stays in place, the system will continue to favor rescue intervention over prevention and proactive health. No amount of exhortation can change that. What the system cannot price, it cannot sustain.

Before proposing alternatives—whether

market-based, technology-enabled, or outcome-linked—we must first see clearly what the current system is designed to do. Only then can we ask a more constructive question: not how to work harder within the existing rules, but whether those rules still make sense in a world where health is shaped over decades, not moments.

Chapter 2: The Currency of Medicine

Every pricing system reflects the conditions under which it was built.

The RVU system emerged in a world where medical knowledge was scarce and slow to change. There were few authoritative texts, no shared digital records, and no reliable way to compare experience across institutions. Conferences were accessible to a small professional elite. Most learning occurred through apprenticeship and personal mentorship, passed down case by case rather than tested across populations. Expertise accumulated slowly and unevenly, and much of what mattered could not be verified outside the individual practitioner.

In that context, experience-based judgment was scarce. It lived inside people. It took years—often decades—to acquire. A neurosurgeon, cardiac surgeon, or trauma surgeon was valuable not simply because of the procedure performed, but because of the accumulated judgment behind it: when to act, how to act, and how to respond when things went wrong. Each new practitioner began largely from scratch.

The payment system reflected that reality. What it was really pricing was not the procedure alone, but the scarcity of experience behind it.

The Relative Value Unit, or RVU, was a pragmatic solution to a practical problem. Policymakers needed a way to pay physicians consistently under Medicare. Charges varied widely. Prices bore little relationship to effort. There was no common measure that allowed one kind of medical work to be compared to another.

RVUs provided that measure. Each billable service was assigned a relative value meant to reflect physician effort, practice costs, and risk. Once those values were set, they could be converted into payment using a standard formula. RVUs became the internal currency of the system.

At the time, this approach made sense. Medicine was dominated by acute illness. Work was episodic. Most services could be described as discrete events. The RVU framework fit the clinical reality of the era.

It also carried an institutional advantage. By framing payment as a technical exercise, it moved decisions about value out of open debate and into professional committees. Pricing could be described as neutral, data-driven, and expert rather than political.

Over time, this technical solution hardened into infrastructure.

RVUs were written into contracts. Compensation plans were built around them. Productivity came to be measured in units generated rather than risk reduced or health preserved. Health systems learned to manage by spreadsheet. Physicians learned to track their worth in currency that rewarded volume over trajectory.

What began as a measuring tool became a governing system.

For a while, the distortions were manageable. But the assumptions that justified the system began to erode.

Medical knowledge no longer accumulates slowly or privately. It changes rapidly and propagates widely. Learning is shared, updated, and refined across populations. Pattern recognition does not reset with each new practitioner.

A modern surgical robot does not begin its first case as a novice. It arrives carrying the experience of thousands of prior procedures performed across a network. Each new case refines the model for the next. The learning curve that once justified high procedural pricing is no longer owned by any single human.

The system, however, continues to pay as if it were.

By 2026, the assumptions that underpinned this pricing structure no longer hold. The RVU framework was built to price individual memory and episodic action. It cannot adapt to a world in which knowledge is shared, learning is continuous, and expertise is replicated at scale. No incremental adjustment can change that.

This creates a profound mispricing. Execution continues to command a premium even as much of the underlying knowledge becomes non-rival and repeatable. What grows scarce instead is judgment about whether to intervene at all, trust that sustains adherence over time, and accountability for the trajectory of health rather than the success of a single event.

The failure of the system is often misunderstood as a failure of professionalism. It is not. Clinicians respond rationally to the rules under which they work. A pricing system that pays reliably for intervention and poorly for upstream judgment will, over time, favor the former. Moral appeals cannot overcome rent, payroll, and institutional survival.

Nor is nostalgia a solution. The image of the wise generalist providing reassurance at the front door of the system once served a purpose. In a world of limited knowledge, experience compensated for uncertainty. But outdated upstream judgment—uninformed by current evidence or distorted by personal bias—is not benign. It can delay diagnosis, obscure risk, and cause harm. Familiarity is not value.

The deeper problem is that the system lacks a way to distinguish good judgment from bad. RVUs can count visits. They can count procedures. They cannot reliably price discernment, nor can they tell the difference between guidance that reduces risk and reassurance that merely feels comforting.

This limitation becomes more consequential as upstream intervention grows more effective. The system continues to reward late rescue while lacking a credible way to pay for the work that prevents problems from arising—or for the responsibility required to guide health across time.

At this point, the persistence of the RVU system is no longer a technical puzzle. It is an institutional one.

When the rules governing health payment are set primarily by those whose livelihoods depend on the existing structure, the outcome is predictable. This is not a charge of bad faith. It is a recognition of human incentives. Pricing health in a modern society requires broader and more independent stewardship than closed-door committees of interested parties can reasonably provide.

RVUs solved yesterday's problem. They now stand in the way of solving tomorrows.

Chapter 3: What Medical Work Is Worth

Every pricing system depends on governance.

Someone decides what counts as medical work, how it is measured, and what it is worth. Those decisions shape behavior more reliably than mission statements, ethics codes, or professional ideals. In medicine, where payment determines which activities survive and which disappear, governance is not a side issue. It is the system.

In the United States, much of this authority rests with a little-known body called the Relative Value Scale Update Committee, or RUC. Convened by the American Medical Association, the RUC brings together representatives from medical specialty societies to recommend how billable medical services should be valued.

The committee's work is technical by design. It reviews surveys, estimates time and effort, and proposes relative values for new or revised billing codes. Its recommendations are transmitted to the federal government, which adopts the vast majority of them as the basis for Medicare payment.

This arrangement is often defended as practical. Who better to judge medical work, the argument goes, than physicians themselves? Expertise should guide valuation. Politics should stay out.

In the historical context in which the RUC emerged, this logic had force. Medical work was difficult to observe from the outside. Knowledge was specialized. Judgment was embodied in individuals and learned through apprenticeship. Allowing professionals to advise on value seemed reasonable.

Over time, however, an advisory role hardened into de facto authority.

Because Medicare payment shapes the entire health economy, RUC recommendations influence far more than federal spending. Commercial insurers follow Medicare's lead. Health systems build compensation models around its values. Training pathways adjust to what pays. The RUC does not merely advise the system. It governs it.

The composition of that governing body therefore matters. Specialty societies representing procedure-based fields hold substantial influence. This reflects history and structure, not conspiracy. Procedural medicine expanded rapidly during the decades when the RUC took shape. Those specialties organized early and effectively. Their representatives now occupy much of the decision-making space.

The result is predictable. Work that resembles the experience of those in the room is easier to describe, easier to defend, and easier to value. Work that is diffuse, longitudinal, preventive, or population-based is harder to specify and easier to discount.

Public health never meaningfully entered this valuation framework because it never had a seat at the table where medical work was priced. Its contributions—risk reduction, early detection, environmental intervention—do not fit neatly into episode-based billing. Lacking representation and lacking a compatible unit of account, it remained peripheral to the payment system, regardless of its impact on health outcomes.

This exclusion did not require malice. It required only structural omission.

No group of professionals, however capable or well intentioned, can be expected to neutrally redesign a system that determines their income. This is not a moral failing. It is a predictable feature of human incentives. When governance is dominated by interested parties, the range of imaginable change narrows.

As medicine has changed, this governance model has not.

Chronic disease now dominates morbidity and cost. Health increasingly depends on early intervention, sustained guidance, and coordination across time. Digital tools allow monitoring and pattern recognition far beyond the clinic. Yet the valuation apparatus remains anchored to an older conception of work, one centered on discrete, billable events.

The consequences are not abstract. Over the past several decades, clinicians across the country have developed rigorous, evidence-based approaches to reducing risk, coordinating chronic illness, and intervening earlier—often with better outcomes and lower long-term cost. Many of these innovations failed not because they lacked merit, but because they could not be translated into billable units. Without a way to be paid, even the best ideas could not survive.

The system did not reject these approaches explicitly. It simply starved them.

Attempts to reform the structure from within have repeatedly stalled. New billing codes proliferate without altering priorities. Pilot programs demonstrate promise but struggle to scale. Incremental adjustments are absorbed while the center of gravity remains fixed.

This persistence is often mistaken for stability. It is better understood as inertia.

When a pricing system no longer reflects the realities it governs, stewardship must change. That does not mean excluding clinicians from valuation. It means broadening the table and modernizing the framework. Patients, employers, public payers, technologists, and independent analysts all have stakes in how health work is priced. So do future clinicians, whose training will follow whatever the system rewards.

Pricing health in the twenty-first century requires sobriety. It requires recognizing conflicts of interest without demonizing them. It requires separating expertise from authority. And it requires institutions capable of valuing work that unfolds over years rather than moments.

The question, then, is not whether the current governance model once worked. It did. The question is whether it can guide a system whose core challenges have changed.

It cannot.

Chapter 4: Why Prevention Struggles to Survive in a Rescue-Based Economy

Prevention is widely praised and poorly rewarded.

Nearly every health policy document, corporate mission statement, and professional oath endorses the idea of intervening early. Yet year after year, resources continue to flow toward late rescue. The explanation is not hypocrisy. It is structure.

Prevention does not fail because it lacks evidence. It fails because it lacks a business model.

In a system governed by episodic payment, value is assigned to events. A test, a procedure, an admission—these can be coded, priced, and reimbursed. Prevention, by contrast, is defined by what does not happen. A stroke avoided. A complication never seen. A crisis that fails to materialize. These outcomes are real, but they do not announce themselves in ways the billing system can recognize.

The result is a quiet asymmetry. Rescue produces visible activity. Prevention produces absence. One generates claims. The other generates silence.

This asymmetry shapes behavior long before intent enters the picture. Health systems build capacity around what pays reliably. Investors fund technologies that fit the existing payment rails. Clinicians are trained to work efficiently within short encounters because that is where compensation is anchored. Prevention survives only when it can be attached to rescue or subsidized by it.

This is why preventive work is so often fragmented. Risk is identified in one place, addressed in another, and followed—if at all—somewhere else. Responsibility dissolves between visits. No one owns the trajectory, because ownership is not paid for.

Attempts to correct this imbalance typically take one of two forms. The first is exhortation. Physicians are encouraged to "focus more on prevention." Patients are urged to "take responsibility for their health." Employers are asked to "invest upstream." These appeals assume that motivation is the missing ingredient.

It is not.

The second approach is to bolt preventive measures onto the existing structure. Quality metrics are layered onto fee-for-service payment. Bonuses are offered for meeting targets. New codes are introduced for counseling or screening. These measures produce modest improvements, but they do not change the underlying economics. Prevention remains marginal because it remains dependent.

The deeper problem is that prevention unfolds over time, while the payment system resets at each encounter. The work that reduces long-term risk—monitoring, adjustment, coaching, coordination—does not fit cleanly into short billing cycles. It requires continuity, not throughput.

This is where innovation repeatedly runs aground.

Over the past several decades, clinicians and researchers have developed sophisticated approaches to managing chronic disease, reducing cardiovascular risk, preventing complications, and supporting behavior change. Many of these approaches work. Some dramatically reduce downstream intervention. Yet few scale.

The reason is consistent. When prevention succeeds, it reduces the volume of billable rescue. Under the prevailing payment model, success undermines revenue. The system responds rationally by limiting adoption.

This creates a paradox. Innovations that promise to reduce cost and improve health are treated as financial threats. Technologies that optimize late intervention are welcomed because they generate billable activity. The system learns, implicitly, which kinds of innovation are safe.

The consequences extend beyond economics. Clinicians experience frustration as they watch preventable problems escalate. Patients encounter a system that reacts forcefully once crisis arrives but remains passive beforehand. Employers absorb rising costs without seeing corresponding gains in workforce health.

None of this requires cynicism to explain. It requires only attention to incentives.

As long as payment is tied to events

rather than trajectories, prevention will struggle to survive. As long as responsibility ends when the visit ends, no one will be accountable for what happens in between. As long as success is defined as activity rather than avoided harm, rescue will dominate.

This is not a failure of intention. It is a failure of design.

A system that wishes to move upstream must be able to recognize upstream work. It must be able to pay for judgment exercised early, trust built over time, and accountability sustained across years rather than minutes. Without a way to value these activities explicitly, prevention will remain an aspiration rather than an operating principle.

The problem is now visible. Costs continue to rise. Chronic disease consumes resources. Innovation accelerates but bends toward late intervention. The question is no longer whether prevention matters. The question is whether the system is capable of supporting it.

Answering that requires a different way of thinking about value.

Chapter 5: What The American System Asks of Clinicians—and What It Takes Away

Every pricing system carries an implicit job description.

In American medicine, that job description is rarely stated plainly. It emerges instead through schedules, metrics, and compensation plans. Over time, clinicians learn what is expected of them not from mission statements, but from what is counted.

The prevailing system asks clinicians to do two incompatible things at once. They are expected to act as stewards of health—exercising judgment, earning trust, and guiding people across time—while being paid as producers of billable events. These roles pull in opposite directions.

The tension is not subtle.

Clinicians are trained to notice early signals, to weigh uncertainty, and to intervene thoughtfully. Yet they are scheduled in ways that discourage deliberation. They are held responsible for outcomes they do not control, while being compensated for activity they do. They are urged to practice prevention in systems that reward rescue.

Over time, adaptation sets in.

Visits shorten. Documentation expands. Attention shifts from the person to the screen. Decisions are shaped less by what would be best upstream and more by what fits the available slot. None of this requires cynicism. It is a rational response to structural pressure.

The language used to describe this experience often misses the point. Burnout is framed as an individual failing—a matter of resilience, balance, or mindset. Wellness programs are offered. Mindfulness apps proliferate.

These interventions assume that the problem lies within the clinician.

It does not.

Burnout is better understood as moral compression. Clinicians are asked to care about outcomes they are not given the time, tools, or authority to influence. They are held accountable for trajectories they are not paid to manage. The result is frustration, detachment, and, eventually, withdrawal.

The system also distorts professional identity.

Training pathways increasingly align with what pays. Procedural specialties expand. Cognitive and longitudinal roles struggle to recruit. Young clinicians learn early which forms of work are respected and which are treated as overhead. The message is absorbed quietly but clearly.

Innovation follows the same pattern. Clinicians who develop new approaches to risk reduction, coordination, or early intervention often do so at personal cost. Their work may improve outcomes and reduce downstream intervention, but without a way to be paid, it remains fragile. Many promising models dissolve when grant funding ends or leadership changes.

The system does not reject these efforts explicitly. It simply fails to sustain them.

This creates a narrowing of professional possibility. Clinicians who might otherwise devote their careers to upstream work learn that doing so requires cross-subsidization, personal sacrifice, or institutional protection. Those options are not available to most.

The effect compounds across generations. Training adapts to the system as it exists, not as it ought to be. Skills that cannot be billed are de-emphasized. Judgment exercised over time becomes harder to teach because it becomes harder to practice.

None of this implies that clinicians are powerless. It does imply that professionalism alone cannot overcome structural misalignment. A system that asks clinicians to act as stewards of health while paying them as producers of volume will continue to exhaust them.

This exhaustion has consequences beyond morale. It affects decision-making, continuity, and trust. Patients sense when guidance is rushed or fragmented. Clinicians sense when their role has been reduced to throughput. The relationship frays on both sides.

At this point, the question is no longer whether clinicians should adapt. They already have. The question is whether the system can evolve to support the kind of work it claims to value.

Answering that requires more than compassion. It requires redesign.

Chapter 6: Why Innovation Fails to Scale — It Threatens Revenue

American medicine does not lack innovation.

New technologies emerge each year. Data grows richer. Algorithms improve. Clinical insight deepens. Yet despite this constant activity, the system itself changes very little. Costs rise. Outcomes improve unevenly. The same frustrations recur.

The reason is not mystery. Innovation does not fail because it is poorly designed. It fails because it is introduced into a system that cannot absorb it.

Every innovation enters a set of rails: payment rules, governance structures, and professional incentives. These rails determine whether an idea spreads, stalls, or quietly disappears. No matter how promising the innovation, it must fit the existing logic to survive.

In American medicine, that logic is episodic payment.

Innovations that optimize rescue fit easily. A faster scanner. A better device. A more precise intervention. These tools enhance what the system already pays for. They generate billable events. They are welcomed, adopted, and scaled.

Innovations that reduce the need for rescue face a different fate.

Tools that detect risk earlier, guide behavior over time, or prevent deterioration often demonstrate impressive results. They reduce hospitalizations. They avert complications. They smooth trajectories. But because they diminish the volume of billable events, they undermine revenue. The system responds rationally by limiting their reach.

This pattern repeats across domains.

Remote monitoring programs show promise, then stall. Chronic disease management models deliver results, then fade. Multidisciplinary coordination efforts improve outcomes, then dissolve when grant funding ends. The failure mode is consistent: no durable payment mechanism emerges to support the work once novelty wears off.

Innovation becomes a pilot, not a platform.

This creates a distorted landscape. Entrepreneurs learn quickly which kinds of ideas are safe. Technologies that enhance documentation, billing efficiency, or procedural throughput attract capital. Tools that replace or reduce encounters struggle to find buyers, even when they improve health.

Clinicians experience this distortion

firsthand. Those who develop new approaches to upstream intervention often do so at personal or institutional risk. Their work may succeed clinically while failing economically. Without a way to be paid, sustainability depends on goodwill rather than design.

The problem is often misdiagnosed as a technology gap. The assumption is that better tools will eventually force change. History suggests otherwise.

Technology does not override pricing. Pricing governs technology.

As long as the payment system rewards events rather than trajectories, innovation will continue to bend toward late intervention. New tools will be repurposed to support old priorities. Progress will accumulate at the margins while the core remains unchanged.

This is why repeated waves of innovation produce similar disappointment. Each new generation of tools promises transformation. Each encounters the same constraints. The wall is structural.

There is also a deeper tension at work.

As artificial intelligence advances, it absorbs more pattern recognition and procedural knowledge. Tasks that once required extensive human experience become standardized, replicable, and scalable. Execution improves. Precision increases. Costs per intervention fall.

Yet the system continues to pay as if value still resides primarily in execution.

This mismatch intensifies the collision. Innovation makes intervention cheaper and more effective, while pricing continues to reward it disproportionately. Meanwhile, the human work that remains essential—judgment under uncertainty, trust-building, accountability over time—remains difficult to price and therefore difficult to sustain.

The result is a paradox. The more capable technology becomes, the less aligned the payment system grows with actual sources of value.

At this stage, the question is not whether innovation should continue. It will. The question is whether innovation alone can fix a system whose economic signals point in the wrong direction.

It cannot.

A pricing system built for episodic action will continue to pull innovation back toward episodic use. Without a new way to value longitudinal responsibility and upstream judgment, even the most powerful tools will be constrained.

Innovation stalls because a pricing system built to pay for events cannot sustain tools that reduce the need for those events. As long as medical work is valued primarily at the moment of intervention, advances that move risk upstream will continue to collide with the same wall. The constraint is not technological. It is economic.

Chapter 7: What Humans Still Do Better Than Machines

Every major technological shift forces a revaluation of human work.

When machines take over tasks that were once scarce, expensive, or slow, the question is not whether humans become irrelevant. The question is which forms of human effort remain essential—and therefore worth paying for.

Medicine has reached that point.

Artificial intelligence now excels at pattern recognition across large data sets. It can detect correlations, flag anomalies, and compare a single case to millions of others in real time. Robotics improves precision and consistency. Automation reduces error in repeatable tasks. These advances are real, durable, and accelerating.

They change the economics of execution.

What once required years of repetition to master can now be assisted, guided, or standardized. Technical skill no longer resets with each practitioner. Knowledge accumulates collectively and propagates instantly. The value of individual memory declines as shared systems improve.

This does not diminish medicine. It clarifies it.

As machines absorb execution and recognition, the remaining human work becomes more visible.

That work is not mystery. It is judgment.

Judgment is the ability to choose under uncertainty when evidence is incomplete, values conflict, or outcomes cannot be fully predicted. It involves deciding whether to act at all, not merely how to act. Machines can inform these decisions, but they cannot own them.

Closely related is trust.

Trust is not compliance. It is voluntary alignment over time. People follow guidance when they believe it is offered in their interest and adapted to their circumstances. Trust is earned through consistency, honesty, and presence—not through accuracy alone.

The third human function is accountability.

Accountability, in this context, does not mean blame. It means sustained responsibility for a trajectory rather than a moment. It means someone stands with a person across time, adjusts guidance as conditions change, and does not disappear between episodes.

Together, these three functions—judgment, trust, and accountability—

define the human role in modern medicine.

They are also precisely the functions the current pricing system fails to recognize.

Judgment exercised early prevents unnecessary intervention later. Trust reduces friction, improves adherence, and smooths decision-making. Accountability keeps risk from drifting unnoticed. Each of these activities reduces billable events. Each therefore struggles to survive in a system that pays for events.

This creates a widening gap between where value is generated and where payment is directed.

The more capable machines become, the more expensive this gap grows. As execution improves and costs fall, the system continues to reward it disproportionately. Meanwhile, the work that determines whether execution is needed at all remains undervalued.

This inversion is not sustainable.

It also exposes a false choice that has lingered in debates about technology and medicine. The question is not whether machines will replace clinicians. They will not. The question is whether the system will pay humans for the work machines cannot do.

A system that continues to price execution while neglecting judgment will misuse both. Machines will be deployed late rather than early. Humans will be rushed rather than deliberate. Outcomes will improve at the margins while costs continue to rise.

Recognizing uniquely human work is therefore not an ethical gesture. It is an economic necessity.

Any future pricing system must be able to distinguish between execution and stewardship. It must recognize work that unfolds over time rather than at a point. And it must align payment with responsibility rather than throughput.

Technology makes this possible. It also makes delay more costly.

The work of humans in medicine has not disappeared. It has moved upstream. The system has yet to follow.

Chapter 8: When the Market Moves On

Every pricing system eventually confronts reality.

For much of modern medical history, American health care has been insulated from ordinary market signals. Prices were opaque. Demand was mediated. Payment was buffered by employers and governments. The system could drift without immediate consequence.

That insulation is eroding.

What many incumbents feel today is not panic, but recognition. A quiet sense that something fundamental has shifted—and that no one with authority has quite said it out loud. Utilization patterns are changing. Margins are compressing. Upstream intervention is becoming more effective. And the old assumptions no longer feel secure.

The most common fear voiced about technology in medicine is that machines will replace clinicians. This fear is understandable—and largely misplaced. Technology is not taking clinicians' jobs. What it is doing is revealing a mismatch between what the system pays for and what people increasingly want to pay for.

That distinction matters.

Automation does not displace work that remains scarce. It displaces work that has become routine. When execution improves, spreads, and becomes replicable, its price falls. This is not ideology. It is how markets behave.

For decades, execution was scarce. Technical skill accumulated slowly. Judgment lived in individuals. Experience could not be copied or shared at scale. Paying a premium for intervention made sense.

That world no longer exists.

Today, procedural knowledge is standardized, assisted, and continuously refined. Systems learn collectively. Outcomes improve as repetition scales. What once justified high prices—the scarcity of experience—has diminished.

The pricing system, however, has not kept pace.

It continues to value intervention as if it were still rare, individualized, and non-transferable. Meanwhile, the work that increasingly determines outcomes—early judgment, sustained guidance, and responsibility over time—remains poorly priced or unpaid.

This creates growing resistance. Patients prefer earlier answers and fewer crises. Employers look for predictability rather than episodic shock. Governments search for sustainability rather than heroics. These preferences are not ideological. They are practical.

In this sense, displacement is not imposed. It is chosen.

Clinicians and institutions that insist on being paid primarily for work that no longer requires uniquely human judgment will not find themselves without tasks. They will find themselves with fewer buyers willing to pay premium prices for those tasks.

This is not a warning. It is a description.

The central risk facing incumbents is therefore not automation. It is mispricing. A system that continues to reward late intervention while neglecting upstream stewardship will quietly shrink the role of those who cling to the old valuation—not through confrontation, but through preference.

The alternative is not resistance. It is redesign.

Human work in medicine remains essential. But its value has moved upstream. It now lies in deciding whether to intervene, earning trust over time, and remaining accountable for trajectories rather than moments. If payment does not follow that shift, the market will adjust without coordination or intent.

This shift is not abstract. It is being driven by artificial intelligence. AI collapses learning curves, standardizes execution, and makes pattern recognition cheap. Work that once justified premium pricing because it was scarce no longer is. This is not a future scenario. It is the present condition under which health markets are already adjusting.

Technology has already moved. Preferences are following.

The only remaining question is whether the pricing system will adapt deliberately—or be bypassed.

Chapter 9: The Downstream Rescue Health Economy—and What Happens When It Shrinks

Modern medicine is not only a clinical enterprise. It is an industrial one.

Over the past half-century, an entire economic ecosystem has grown around late intervention. Hospitals, device manufacturers, imaging companies, staffing firms, revenue-cycle vendors, construction projects, and training pipelines all depend, directly or indirectly, on the volume of downstream activity. The system does not merely respond to illness. It is built to process it.

This structure did not arise by accident. Acute care once represented the clearest, most reliable locus of value. Disease declared itself late. Intervention required infrastructure. Rescue saved lives. Payment followed necessity.

That logic shaped investment.

Hospitals expanded capacity. Device companies refined tools for increasingly precise intervention. Operating rooms multiplied. Business models assumed steady growth in utilization. Training programs adapted to meet demand. An economy formed around crisis management, and for decades it worked.

But economies built around a single assumption become fragile when that assumption changes.

The assumption now under strain is simple: that downstream rescue will continue to be the primary engine of value.

It will not.

Upstream detection, interventionalwithout-surgery techniques, minimally invasive approaches, and continuous monitoring are reducing the need for many forms of late intervention. Some procedures are being displaced entirely. Others are becoming shorter, safer, and less frequent. Lengths of stay shrink. Admissions decline. Margins compress.

This shift is often framed as a technological disruption. It is better understood as a utilization problem.

The system is not losing relevance. It is losing volume.

For institutions built around throughput, this feels existential. Fixed costs remain. Debt obligations persist. Staffing models lag reality. When utilization falls, the response is often defensive: consolidation, pricing pressure, acquisition, or lobbying for protection.

None of this reflects bad faith. It reflects survival.

Hospitals, in particular, sit at the center of this tension. They are essential institutions, but they are optimized for rescue. Their economics assume beds filled, operating rooms booked, and procedures reimbursed. When prevention succeeds, hospitals do not celebrate. They absorb loss.

This creates a structural conflict between what improves population health and what sustains downstream institutions.

Medical technology companies face a similar reckoning. Devices designed for high-volume procedural use encounter slowing demand as alternatives emerge. Imaging platforms compete for shrinking slices of utilization. Innovation shifts toward efficiency rather than expansion.

Private equity and real estate structures built on predictable procedural flow feel the pressure early. Staffing models strain. Training pipelines misalign. The ecosystem tightens.

Pharmaceutical companies, by contrast, experience a different trajectory. Many already operate upstream. They price long-term risk modification, not episodic intervention. Their incentives align more naturally with chronic disease management and prevention. This distinction matters.

The problem, then, is not medicine versus technology, or clinicians versus machines. It is that an entire downstream economy is organized around a form of value that is becoming less central.

This does not mean downstream institutions disappear. It means their role must change.

The future is not a world without hospitals or intervention. It is a world with fewer crises, later interventions, and higher thresholds for rescue. Downstream capacity will still matter—but it will no longer define growth.

The danger lies in denial.

If downstream institutions attempt to preserve volume by resisting upstream progress, they will fail. Utilization will fall regardless. If they attempt to extract higher prices for diminishing value, resistance will intensify. Employers, governments, and patients will seek alternatives.

The opportunity lies in transition.

Hospitals can become anchors of continuity rather than endpoints of crisis. Device companies can pivot toward tools that support early decision-making, monitoring, and minimally invasive care. Health systems can reorganize around longitudinal responsibility rather than episodic throughput. Training can adapt to new roles.

But this transition requires one thing above all: a pricing system that no longer treats prevention as a threat.

As long as payment rewards rescue volume, downstream institutions will experience upstream success as financial harm. As long as that tension persists, resistance is rational.

This is why payment reform is not a side issue. It is the keystone.

A system that pays for judgment, trust, and accountability upstream allows downstream institutions to reposition themselves without collapse. It turns prevention from a liability into a revenue stream. It creates room for redesign rather than retrenchment.

Absent that change, the downstream economy will shrink anyway—unevenly, painfully, and without coordination.

The choice is not between protecting the old system and embracing the new. The choice is between managed transition and unmanaged decline.

Health care continues to become more expensive not because tools to reduce cost are lacking, but because the pricing system rewards late intervention and penalizes anything that reduces the need for it.

Chapter 10: Pricing What Matters

Every pay system reveals what it values. In health, the signal has long been clear. Value appears when something breaks. Payment follows the fix. The more complex and visible the intervention, the higher the reward.

That logic once matched reality. It no longer does.

Artificial intelligence has changed what work is scarce and what work is common. Pattern recognition is no longer rare. Repetition is no longer costly. Knowledge no longer resets with each practitioner. What once took years to learn can now be supported, checked, and improved at scale.

Pricing has not caught up.

This is not a coming problem. It is a present one. The question is no longer whether health will be repriced. It is whether repricing happens on purpose, with design and retraining, or later, through delay and attrition. If pricing does not change, roles will still change. They will simply do so without preparation, without fairness, and without choice.

The central flaw in today's system is not technical. It is structural. Payment is tied to moments rather than paths. A moment is a visit, a scan, a cut, a stay. A path is the course of a person's health over time: whether risk is seen early or late, whether signals are acted on or ignored, whether decisions are made before damage hardens, and whether anyone remains responsible once the moment has passed.

Health is shaped by paths. Payment remains fixed on moments

A system built around moments cannot reward early judgment. It cannot support steady guidance. It cannot pay for staying responsible between crises. Those actions reduce later intervention, and under current rules, reducing intervention reduces revenue. This is why health care grows more expensive even as tools capable of lowering cost improve. The system is paid to act late and penalized for acting early. AI does not cause this problem. It makes it visible.

AI draws a hard line between work that needs humans and work that does not. Tasks that follow rules, repeat often, or rely on matching patterns are now cheap and fast. The price of that work falls. What remains scarce is work that requires choice.

Choice means deciding when not to act. It means weighing risk before harm declares itself. It means knowing when to wait and when to move and standing behind that decision when facts are incomplete. That work cannot be copied, rushed, or done once. It unfolds over time. If it is not paid for, it disappears.

Judgment is not instinct. It is trained decision-making under uncertainty. In health, judgment matters most early, when options still exist. Once damage is done, choice narrows and cost rises. A sane pricing system treats judgment as real work. It pays for thinking, checking, adjusting, and deciding across time, not for the number of actions taken. Other fields already do this. Health has resisted because it tied value to visible acts. AI removes that excuse.

Trust has been treated as sentiment. It is not. Trust is what allows guidance to work before crisis. People act on advice when it fits their lives and when someone remains present after it is given. Trust lowers cost by preventing delay. It cannot be built in a rush. A system that wants trust must pay for continuity and follow-through. If it does not, trust remains incidental rather than structural.

Responsibility is rarer still. Responsibility means owning the path, not just the step. It means risk is noticed rather than handed off. It means someone is accountable when nothing urgent is happening. Today, no one is paid for this. Responsibility is split across visits and sites. Harm looks sudden only because no one was paid to see it forming. A future pricing system must name responsibility and pay for it directly, or it will not exist.

None of this end's intervention. It changes its place. When early work is paid for, fewer people reach crisis. Intervention becomes rarer and more exact. When it is needed, it matters more. Fewer interventions do not signal failure. They signal success upstream.

This shift lowers cost because it changes timing. Late work is expensive. Early work is not, but only if it is paid for. Right now, early work shrinks because it is unpaid, while late work grows because it is rewarded. AI widens this gap by making late work faster and cheaper while leaving early work invisible. Repricing closes the gap.

The tools to support this already exist. Continuous data, shared records, pattern alerts, AI support. What is missing is not capability but will.

Health will be repriced. AI has already made that unavoidable. The remaining choice is whether repricing is done deliberately, with design and retraining, or indirectly, through delay and attrition. There is no third option.

Chapter 11: The New Human Work

Patients have never had autonomy in any meaningful sense. Late-stage medicine is coercive by nature. When disease has hardened, options have narrowed, and urgency dominates, choice exists only on paper. Consent is obtained, but agency is gone. Decisions are made under fear, time pressure, and unequal knowledge. Autonomy was never a governing value in health because the system was not built to support it.

That condition has changed.

Upstream diagnosis, continuous interpretation, and sustained responsibility alter the nature of decision-making itself. When people understand risk before damage sets in, when guidance is ongoing rather than episodic, and when responsibility is owned across time, decisions are made under conditions that allow real choice. Autonomy becomes possible not because more options are offered, but because decisions occur before fate closes them.

Doctor AI and Health 4.0 do not promise better decisions at the end. They make decision-making possible before the end arrives. This is not an ethical refinement. It is a structural change in power.

That shift also changes human work.

Some work is shrinking. Tasks built on repetition, routine execution, or control of information lose value as AI spreads. Roles that exist because knowledge was once scarce or access was guarded come under pressure. This does not mean those roles vanish overnight. It does mean they no longer anchor long-term careers.

Other work grows because it remains hard.

Early decision-making grows because cost and outcome are shaped long before intervention. Someone must weigh weak signals, judge risk before damage, and decide when to act and when to wait. AI can inform that work, but it cannot own it. That authority remains human, and it matters more now than it did before.

Sustained guidance grows because health does not move in straight lines. Plans change. Conditions shift. People need steady interpretation rather than one-time advice. This work depends on trust and lowers cost precisely because it keeps trouble from escalating. It has always existed. It has rarely been paid for.

Escalation authority grows because someone must decide when restraint ends and action begins. This work replaces reflex with judgment and spreads accountability back to where it belongs. As machines handle more execution, this authority becomes more valuable, not less.

These forms of work do not expand by accident. They expand only if systems choose to recognize them, train for them, and pay for them. Without that choice, they remain informal and fragile, carried by individuals rather than institutions.

Clinicians are not becoming unnecessary. They are being asked to do different work. The clinician whose value lies in early judgment, sustained guidance, and owned responsibility will be needed. The clinician whose role rests mainly on volume of routine execution will face pressure. This is not a moral claim. It is an economic one.

Responding well requires retraining, not exhortation. It requires redesigned roles, not slogans. It requires payment aligned with responsibility rather than habit. Without those changes, clinicians will absorb the transition privately through overload, burnout, and exit.

For patients, the gain is not comfort. It is agency. Earlier understanding means fewer forced decisions. Continuity means fewer handoffs. Clear responsibility means fewer moments of being told that no one owns the problem. Autonomy becomes real because it arrives before crisis.

For clinicians reading this and thinking, Right — this is true, the question is no longer abstract. It is practical. Which of my skills remain scarce? Which are losing value? Where is judgment protected? Where is responsibility paid for? Environments that rush thinking, fragment responsibility, and add AI without training have already chosen delay. Environments that protect early judgment, invest in retraining, and align pay with responsibility are choosing design.

Change will happen either way. The difference is whether it is shaped early or absorbed later, one person at a time.

Chapter 12: Health Care Leadership

Leadership in health has long been defined by steadiness. The ability to reassure, to maintain continuity, to keep institutions functioning despite strain; these skills have been treated as competence. In a slower world, that approach often worked. In the present one, it no longer does.

The first question leadership now faces is not strategic but intellectual: how honest is our understanding of what is happening?

Across the system, many leaders sense that something fundamental is shifting. They see margins tighten, roles blur, and technology advance faster than governance can respond. Yet few can state clearly what is changing, why it is changing, and what that implies for the work their institutions exist to do. The language remains cautious. The explanations remain partial. The decisions remain deferred.

This raises a harder question: how clear is health leadership, really, about the forces now shaping the system?

Artificial intelligence is no longer a peripheral tool. It is reshaping scarcity itself—what knowledge costs, what judgment requires, and what kinds of work still justify human effort. Yet much of health leadership treats AI as an add-on: a pilot, a vendor relationship, a productivity tool layered onto unchanged roles. Few leaders can explain, in plain terms, how AI alters learning curves, collapses experience-based pricing, or shifts value upstream. Fewer still have grappled with what that means for workforce design, training, and authority.

This gap in understanding matters, because leaders who do not grasp the nature of the change cannot guide others through it.

The question then becomes uncomfortable: what do health leaders actually know about AI—not in slogans, but in substance? Do they understand where it replaces human labor, where it amplifies it, and where it exposes mispricing rather than inefficiency? Or are they relying on advisors, vendors, and abstractions to stand in for understanding they do not themselves possess?

Leadership without comprehension becomes delay with a title.

The consequences of that delay are not evenly distributed. They fall hardest on those with the least power to adapt quietly: trainees, early-career clinicians, and staff whose roles are changing without being named. These groups are told to prepare for a future that leadership itself has not defined. They are trained for jobs that may not exist, assessed on metrics that may soon lose relevance, and reassured with language that obscures rather than clarifies.

This raises another question leadership rarely asks openly: how honest are we being with the next generation?

If autonomy is only now becoming structurally possible, if upstream judgment is only now becoming legible and pay-able, then training built around episodic throughput, and late intervention is already misaligned. To continue teaching as if the old system will persist is not neutrality. It is misdirection.

The failure here is not individual. It is systemic. Leadership structures in health, reward continuity of tone more than clarity of thought. They favor consensus over comprehension. They are too much in the day-to-day noise of healthcare to look up at the bigger picture. They produce leaders who are highly skilled at managing institutions as they are, but les equipped to redesign them as they must become.

This is why so many leaders appear suspended in place—experienced, capable, and increasingly at the eye of the storm of change. Many are committed, highly intelligent, with good intent, but because the system that shaped them did not require the skills now demanded, they are behind the curve of learning, and therefore of leading. The result is a kind of institutional stasis: not corruption, but immobilization.

Leadership cannot remain defined by reassurance. It must be defined by understanding, candor, and responsibility.

The leaders of health institutions and those that aspire to leadership now requires they understand and can clearly articulate how AI changes value, not just deploy tools. They must understand pricing as architecture, not accounting. They must be able to say which work is shrinking and which is growing, and to build paths between the two before attrition does that work instead. They must be willing to tell trainees the truth early, while choice still exists.

Anything less transfers the cost of ignorance downward.

This is not a call for disruption. It is a call for intellectual honesty. Leadership that cannot name reality cannot claim stewardship. Leadership that delays comprehension delays justice.

The future of health will not be shaped by those who manage change quietly, but by those who understand it clearly enough to design for it and provide the bridge to health.

Chapter 13: What Other Systems Pay For

The failure of American health pricing is often treated as inevitable, as if no alternative has ever existed. That is not true. Other health systems, operating under different constraints, have long paid for work that the American system treats as incidental.

These systems are not models to copy. They have their own failures and limits. But they demonstrate a simple fact: fee-for-service dominance is not a law of nature, and paying for continuity, judgment, and responsibility is not theoretical.

In the United Kingdom, most physicians are not paid by the act. Hospital doctors are salaried. General practices are paid to care for defined populations, not to generate visits. Payment is detached from volume in ways that make continuity possible, even if imperfect. The system struggles with access and political pressure, but it does not confuse activity with value. A physician's worth is not measured by throughput alone.

In countries such as Norway and the Netherlands, primary care physicians are paid through blended models that combine per-person responsibility with limited fees for service. Patients are listed. Responsibility is explicit. Payment reflects the fact that work unfolds over time rather than at a point. These systems do not eliminate intervention. They place it in context.

South Korea offers a different lesson. It retains fee-for-service payment within universal coverage and has achieved impressive access and efficiency. But it also demonstrates the limits of fee-for-service itself. Volume pressure persists. Prevention remains underweighted. Coverage alone does not solve mispricing.

The point of these comparisons is not superiority. It is feasibility.

Other systems already pay for work that

the American system treats as optional. They pay for continuity because they must. They pay for responsibility because someone has to own the path. They do not pretend that episodic billing can support longitudinal health. What they lack, often, is scale, flexibility, or speed. What they demonstrate is that repricing health is possible without destroying professionalism or agency.

The United States now faces a different opportunity. Artificial intelligence makes upstream judgment, continuous interpretation, and owned responsibility visible and measurable in ways those systems could not achieve when they were designed. The barrier is no longer technical. It is institutional.

Comparative systems show that the American failure is not human. It is structural.

Chapter 14: The System That Makes This Possible

Repricing health requires more than good intentions. It requires structure.

A system built to pay for judgment, trust, and responsibility must be able to see work that unfolds over time. It must be able to distinguish early decision-making from late reaction. It must support continuity without turning clinicians into clerks. Without infrastructure, repricing collapses back into aspiration.

This is where Doctor AI and Health 4.0 enter—not as products, but as conditions

Doctor AI is not a replacement for clinicians. It is the intelligence layer that makes upstream work legible. It aggregates signals across time, surfaces risk before harm declares itself, and supports judgment rather than substituting for it. It carries memory so humans do not have to. It makes responsibility possible without heroics.

Health 4.0 is not a brand. It is a way of organizing care around paths rather than moments. It assumes continuous interpretation rather than episodic reaction. It treats autonomy as something that must be enabled structurally, not granted ceremonially at the end.

Together, they form the minimum structure required to support a different pricing logic.

Without this structure, attempts to pay for upstream work fail. Judgment remains invisible. Trust remains informal. Responsibility remains unpaid. With it, these forms of work become observable, protectable, and pay-able.

This system does not eliminate

intervention. It restores proportion. It allows intervention to arrive later, less often, and with greater effect. It lowers cost not by denial, but by timing.

Most importantly, it changes power.

Patients gain autonomy because decisions occur while choice still exists. Clinicians regain authority because responsibility and judgment are aligned. Leaders regain legitimacy because design replaces delay.

This system does not promise ease. It promises coherence.

Health can now be organized around what actually determines outcomes rather than what merely reacts to failure. That possibility did not exist before. It exists now.

Chapter 15: The Choice

For most of modern medicine, delay was survivable. Knowledge moved slowly, skill was scarce, and late intervention was often, the only option left. Under those conditions, a system built around rescue could persist, even as its costs mounted and its contradictions deepened.

That condition no longer holds.

Artificial intelligence has removed plausible deniability. It has made visible what was once obscured by habit and tradition. It has shown that much of what we pay for arrives after autonomy has already been lost, after options have narrowed, after urgency has replaced choice. At the same time, it has made early judgment, sustained interpretation, and owned responsibility possible at a scale that did not exist before.

This is why the moment matters.

Autonomy was never taken from patients. It was never structurally possible. Decisions made late, under fear and time pressure, are coercive by nature, no matter how carefully consent is obtained. Upstream diagnosis, continuous understanding, and responsibility carried across time change that condition. They make choice possible before fate closes it. That is not a refinement of the existing system. It is a different one.

The same is true for clinicians. Professional authority has eroded not because judgment no longer matters, but because it has been priced out of existence. When thinking is rushed, continuity unpaid, and responsibility fragmented, authority collapses into throughput. Repricing health around what still requires human judgment does not diminish clinicians. It restores coherence between responsibility and power.

Leadership now stands exposed by this shift. Reassurance no longer counts as stewardship. Silence no longer buys time. Delay now transfers cost downward—to trainees prepared for roles that are shrinking, to clinicians absorbing change privately, and to patients facing decisions when choice has already narrowed. Inaction has become a decision, whether acknowledged or not.

None of this requires optimism. It requires honesty.

Health will be repriced. Roles will change. Training will either adapt early or fail late. The only open question is whether this happens deliberately, with design and transition, or indirectly, through delay and attrition.

The tools already exist. The knowledge is already here. What remains undecided is whether those with responsibility will act before responsibility is taken from them by circumstance.

This book has not argued for disruption. It has argued for responsibility in the presence of clarity.

The future of health will be shaped either by people who understand what has changed and choose accordingly, or by systems that refuse to decide and allow attrition to choose for them. That choice is no longer abstract.

The leadership this moment requires does not need to be invented. It already exists within medicine itself—in clinics, emergency departments, intensive care units, classrooms, executive suites, and boardrooms. It lives wherever people are willing to see clearly what is happening and accept responsibility for acting on it.

What is required now is not optimism or reassurance, but clarity and resolve. The willingness to name what work is losing value, to prepare people for work that is gaining it, and to make decisions early enough that choice remains possible. That is how a better health future is delivered—not through slogans, but through clear-eyed judgment applied before delay hardens into fate.

The choices that will shape that future are already being made.